Rebuild & Thrive

Vol. 2

SIMPLE BALANCE EXERCISES TO REGAIN STABILITY AND PREVENT FALL

for Seniors Over 60

DR. HAMRICK NELSON

Disclaimer

The exercises and information presented in this book are designed to promote health, stability, and well-being, particularly for seniors. However, it's important to remember that everyone's body is different, and what works well for one person may not be suitable for another. Before starting any new exercise program, especially if you have any pre-existing medical conditions or concerns, please consult with your doctor or healthcare provider to ensure these routines are safe for you.

While every effort has been made to ensure that the exercises are easy to follow and safe, your health and safety are our top priority. It's important to listen to your body—if you experience any discomfort or pain while performing any exercise, stop immediately and seek guidance from a healthcare professional. This book is intended to be a helpful guide, but it should not replace professional medical advice.

Dr. Hamrick Nelson and the team are committed to your well-being and encourage you to approach these exercises with care, patience, and an understanding of your body's needs.

The goal is to help you live a healthier, more active life, one step at a time.

Table of Contents

ABOUT THE AUTHOR

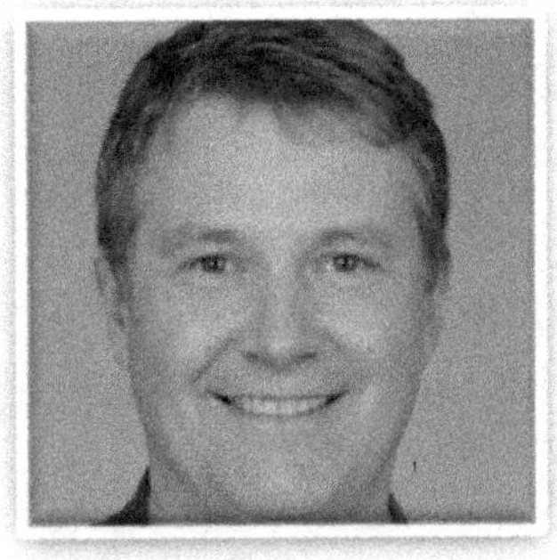 Dr. Hamrick Nelson is a leading voice in fitness and wellness, with a deep passion for helping individuals of all ages live healthier, more active lives. With over two decades of experience in the health and fitness industry, Dr. Nelson has dedicated his career to promoting accessible exercise routines for people at every stage of life. His approach is rooted in the belief that movement is for everyone, regardless of age or physical limitations.

While Dr. Nelson's work spans a wide range of fitness disciplines, he has a special focus on supporting seniors—particularly those over 60. Through his extensive research and hands-on experience, he understands the unique challenges faced by older adults, and he's made it his mission to help them maintain their independence, strength, and vitality. He combines practical knowledge with compassion, creating tailored fitness programs that prioritize safety and long-term health benefits.

Holding advanced degrees in physical therapy and exercise science, Dr. Nelson has worked with countless individuals to enhance their mobility, flexibility, and overall well-being. His books, workshops, and speaking engagements reflect his commitment to helping people of all ages—whether young or senior—stay fit, feel strong, and live life to the fullest.

His program offers an approachable, supportive path to better health, empowering older adults to continue thriving well into their golden years.

INTRODUCTION

There comes a time in life for many of us when we start to notice changes that we never really expected. The way we move, how we feel standing on uneven ground, and even our confidence as we go about our daily routines—all of these tiny changes are linked to one critical factor: balance. Maintaining equilibrium is more than just physical; it is a necessary foundation that allows us to live freely, without the constant fear of stumbling or falling.

I often recall a patient I once had named Orville, a lively man in his early seventies who had retired after decades of working as a landscape photographer. Orville had spent his life traveling around mountains, investigating paths, and photographing nature from perilous vantage points. Despite his physical endurance and agility, age brought about unexpected changes.

The first time I saw Orville, he arrived at our clinic with a small limp and an evident sense of frustration. He stated, almost with defeat, that his balance was no longer what it once was. He described how he stumbled on a patch of damp leaves on his lawn and landed hard on his side. He claimed he was humiliated, not by the fall itself, but by what it signified. "I never used to worry about things like this," he said, slightly surprised.

Orville's experience was a watershed moment, a wake-up call that motivated him to seek solutions. It also made him consider whether balance was something he could actively work on rather than accept as a natural loss with age. He wanted to feel stable and secure again as if he could rely on his body to support him in the same way it had for all those years on the route.

His experience is far from unusual, but it is incredibly significant. For every Orville, countless others are astonished by the minor changes in their bodies throughout time. While aging may cause some unavoidable physical changes, we can nevertheless preserve stability and strength. The road to improved balance may be extremely rewarding—both physically and emotionally. It allows us to reclaim our sense of control and freedom.

This volume was written with these exact situations in mind, and it promises that, like Orville, you, too, may shift your path to better balance, stability, and confidence. This book will walk you through exercises and routines step by step, helping you recapture what you may feel is slipping away: confidence in each stride you take, ease of getting out of a chair, or even the simple joy of moving without hesitation.

This is more than just a book of exercises; it's a guide to understanding the complex interplay between balance, posture, and the body's natural mechanics. In my experience as a health practitioner, I've witnessed firsthand how targeted balance exercises have helped people of all ages, particularly seniors who feel like they're continuously fighting a war with their bodies. The workouts and strategies presented here are intended to be accessible and adaptable—useful to any reader, regardless of current ability level or previous fitness experience.

Much of the framework in this book is intended for gradual advancement. You will not be asked to go immediately into advanced exercises, which is purposeful. Just as Orville confidently progressed from simple seated exercises to standing balances, you'll be encouraged to work at your own pace, focusing on the fundamentals first and then progressing to more difficult moves. There's no rush or deadline. This book is designed to celebrate your path while respecting the speed that feels best for you.

In this book, we'll look at the three main components of balance: *stability, strength, and mindfulness,* and how to use them in safe and sustainable ways. Each segment is constructed around these principles since they serve as the foundation for all of the exercises, movements, and progressions you'll see in the following chapters.

Orville, for example, had a solid foundation of lower-body strength from years of outdoor photography, but over time, he developed certain asymmetries. His hip flexors had tightened from long journeys to remote photography locations, and his ankles had lost mobility from years of climbing with heavy gear. He needs particular activities that attack these imbalances in a slow, safe manner, rather than just "exercise". He had to relearn certain essential practices, such as conscious breathing, careful weight shifts, and basing his motions with awareness, rather than relying solely on his previous habits.

As you progress through this book, you'll see that each exercise plays a specialized role, and each technique has a unique purpose in promoting balance. The goal is to develop the body holistically while also engaging the mind, making each movement an exercise in presence and awareness. This method will help you reconnect with your body in unexpected ways, as well as build confidence as you get more comfortable with each step and stance.

As you proceed through these activities, you will most certainly face hurdles as well as a rising sense of empowerment, just as Orville did. With each chapter, you'll be encouraged to evaluate your progress, understand your body's demands, and make changes that seem appropriate for you.

The workouts are designed to accommodate various levels of ability. Starting with the most basic motions, we'll go over foundational breathing exercises that promote balance and relaxation, then continue to routines geared for beginners, intermediates, and advanced levels. You'll learn how to activate core muscles, increase lower-body strength, and even work on response time—all of which are important components of improving balance and stability.

This book is fundamentally about living with freedom and assurance, not only balance exercises. This book seeks to help you reclaim a sense of independence and trust in your own body, just like Orville did. With consistency, you'll see that these exercises can change not only how you feel physically, but also how you see yourself and the possibilities for your future.

Every step you take in this book is designed to get you closer to that sense of relaxation and security. Whether it's avoiding falls, increasing strength, or simply feeling more connected to each action, the trip ahead is all about regaining your confidence. So, as you begin the first chapter, realize that you are not alone in this journey. Thousands of people have started where you are now, and with each page you turn, you will be laying the groundwork for a lifetime of success.

Let's take the first step together. The route to greater balance, stability, and a brighter future begins here.

CHAPTER 1: RECOGNIZING THE VALUE OF BALANCE FOR SENIORS

A vital component of physical health, balance is frequently disregarded until it starts to decline. For seniors who wish to maintain their independence, self-esteem, and general quality of life, balance is crucial. It is necessary to do everyday tasks, prevent falls, and provide stable mobility. People's balance will gradually deteriorate as they age, but this need not be the case; preserving and improving balance can significantly improve well-being.

The ability of the body to hold itself steadily when moving or staying still is known as balance. A complex interplay between the brain, muscles, joints, and sensory systems including the inner ear and vision keeps this balance. To maintain stability during movement, a person's muscles work in tandem with these sensory inputs. ***The body uses three major systems to keep itself balanced:***

1. ***The Visual System:*** By sending spatial information to the brain, our eyes aid in self-orientation. This includes the locations of objects, people, and buildings in our immediate

environment, which serve as indicators of motion, depth, and distance.

2. ***The Inner Ear:*** It contains the vestibular system, which controls eye movement and balance. It helps us maintain our stability when moving by detecting even minute changes in head position.

3. ***Proprioception:*** This is also referred to as the *"sixth sense,"* enables us to perceive how our limbs and joints move and position themselves. Without looking, you can use this technique to determine the location of each bodily part of the others.

All three systems must cooperate harmoniously for balance to be effective. People's systems naturally alter as they age, making it harder to stay in balance. Among the factors that lead to balance issues in seniors are weakening muscles, decreased joint flexibility, and slowed brain reactions.

As people age, they experience several physiological changes that may impact their ability to balance. Addressing and resolving the problems begins with understanding them.

- Weakness of the Muscles and Bones: Sarcopenia is the aging-related loss of muscular mass. Osteoporosis, which lowers strength and stability, can also be brought on by a decrease in bone density. The body's ability to maintain balance is hampered by weak muscles and bones, particularly when reacting to abrupt changes in direction or posture.

- Reduced Flexibility and Joint Stiffness: As people age, they may experience joint stiffness, which is typically brought on by arthritis or normal wear and tear. Range of motion and flexibility—both necessary for quick adjustments to preserve balance—are restricted by stiffness.

- Slower Reflexes and Reaction Times: As we become older, our reflexes and reaction times go down, which makes it harder to react to possible falls. For instance, it may be more difficult to put one foot forward rapidly when stumbling, which increases the risk of falling.

- Decline of Sensory Functions: People's vision tends to decrease with age, which impacts their ability to balance visually. Additionally, the vestibular system may become less sensitive, which would affect how the body perceives motion and spatial orientation. The body finds it difficult to process environmental information and react correctly when sensory functions are compromised.

The Significance Of Balance In Seniors Daily Lives

Loss of balance directly affects independence and day-to-day functioning. Elderly people who are balanced may walk, bend, turn, reach, and perform other important tasks fearlessly. Here are some ways that balance impacts significant aspects of daily life and why maintaining it is crucial:

1. **Walking and Mobility:** Having a good balance is essential for safe and steady walking. Without it, it could be dangerous to walk on uneven surfaces like grass or sidewalks. Seniors who struggle with balance may steer clear of particular areas or terrain types, which restricts their independence and social opportunities.

2. **Falls and Injury Prevention:** The leading cause of hospitalizations and injuries among the elderly is falling. Falling due to poor balance increases the risk of fractures, bruises, and permanent impairment. Better balance can help reduce falls, which affect one in four people over 65 annually, according to the CDC.

3. **Confidence in Daily Activities:** Confidence deteriorates when equilibrium is upset. It could be difficult to stand up from a seated position, climb stairs, or even just reach for objects on a high shelf. Many elderly people experience a

fear of falling, which can cause them to avoid activities and ultimately result in a reduced quality of life.

4. **Preserving Freedom:** Freedom is a significant aspect of life for many seniors. Cooking, shopping, and household chores all require a certain amount of stability and physical confidence. Seniors with good balance can complete these tasks on their own, maintaining their sense of independence and reducing the need for caregiver assistance.

5. **Joint Health and Posture:** Posture and balance are related. Often, bad posture results from poor balance, which can further strain joints and muscles. This can eventually lead to knee, hip, and back discomfort, which will impede daily function and mobility. Maintaining proper alignment and joint health through good balance lessens the body's wear and tear.

Enhancing equilibrium has benefits that extend beyond the physical world. Exercises involving balance, particularly those performed in groups, have positive social and emotional effects. After taking part in fitness programs that emphasize balance, many seniors say they feel happier, more connected, and more involved. Regular balancing exercises can also enhance mental wellness by:

Increased self-confidence from improved physical stability can reduce anxiety and depression. Seniors who believe they are physically capable are less likely to feel depressed and more likely to participate in social activities.

Exercise, especially balance exercises, has been shown to improve cognitive function in older adults. Proprioceptive and coordination-demanding activities stimulate the brain, perhaps halting cognitive decline.

An essential component of healthy aging is maintaining equilibrium. It affects many everyday actions, including walking and reaching, and is crucial for preserving one's independence and standard of living. Seniors who actively work to improve their balance and understand its significance can increase mobility, reduce their risk of falling, and feel more confident in their day-to-day activities. Balance exercises help seniors live fully, comfortably, and with peace of mind in addition to preventing falls.

The Risk Of Falling

One of the most prevalent and dangerous problems for older adults is falls, which often lead to injuries, a decline in physical capacity, and a loss of independence. Stability and balance may be affected by changes in a person's bone density, joint flexibility, and muscle strength as they age. The likelihood of falling is further increased by health problems, environmental hazards, and adverse drug reactions. The common problems that older adults face and how they raise their risk of falling will be examined in this section. The first step in creating successful preventative strategies is comprehending these barriers.

1. Loss of Strength and Muscle Weakness

As people age, they naturally lose muscle mass and strength, a condition known as sarcopenia. This loss starts in the forties and picks up speed after the age of sixty. For bones and joints to be mobile, stable, and supported, muscles are necessary. Even basic activities like standing, walking, and bending over become more challenging as muscular strength decreases. Elderly people with weak muscles are more likely to fall because they can't quickly restore their posture if they lose their balance.

Apart from sarcopenia, a reduction in physical activity exacerbates muscle weakness. Because of health problems, pain, or a lack of drive, many seniors engage in less physical activity, which contributes to greater muscle loss. This creates a vicious cycle whereby weaker muscles lead to mobility issues, which restrict training potential and hasten the loss of strength.

2. Increased Fragility and Decreased Bone Density

Older adults, especially women, are prone to osteoporosis and reduced bone density. As we age, elements like calcium that give bones their strength are lost. As a result, bones become more brittle, porous, and prone to shattering. In addition to having a higher risk of falling, those with osteoporosis are also more susceptible to fractures, especially those of the wrist, hip, and spine.

Even a small fall could cause serious injuries due to the decreased bone density and strength. For instance, hip fractures are particularly upsetting because they usually lead to long recovery times and a reduced quality of life. As their physical condition deteriorates, seniors may experience a dread of falling, which further restricts their mobility and, regrettably, increases their risk of falling.

3. Decreased Joint Stiffness and Flexibility

Reduced range of motion, stiffness, and discomfort can result from age-related changes in joint health, such as arthritis. For balance, coordination, and fluid movement, joints must be flexible. For instance, although knee and hip mobility are necessary for tasks like standing up from a seated position or climbing stairs, ankle flexibility is essential for balancing when walking on uneven ground.

These movements can be challenging due to stiff or aching joints, which raises the possibility of stumbling, slipping, and making mistakes. Additionally, some seniors may avoid particular positions or actions out of fear of pain, which gradually limits their range of motion. This reduced mobility is a major factor in falls and balance problems.

4. Change in Eyesight and Depth Perception

Vision is crucial for balance because it enables humans to see their surroundings and accurately measure distances. People's ability to perceive depth, peripheral vision, and general clarity all deteriorate with age. Conditions that can significantly impair vision, such as cataracts, glaucoma, macular degeneration, and diabetic retinopathy, are more common in older adults.

Elderly people find it difficult to negotiate obstacles or accurately gauge the height of steps when their depth perception deteriorates. It may be challenging to spot hazards like uneven ground or objects on the floor if you have impaired peripheral vision. For elderly people with vision impairments, poor lighting can make falls more likely, especially at night when they might have to get up to go to the bathroom or move around the house.

5. Side Effects of Medication

For the treatment of chronic conditions such as high blood pressure, diabetes, arthritis, and heart disease, many seniors require numerous drugs. Dizziness, drowsiness, and disorientation are side effects of some medications or drug combinations that affect balance and coordination.

Certain medications, especially those used to treat pain or blood pressure, may make you feel lightheaded or dizzy when you stand up from a sitting position. Elderly people may lose their balance due to orthostatic hypotension, a sudden drop in blood pressure. Seniors who use drugs frequently are more prone to have negative medication interactions. The risks can be reduced by properly managing these drugs and consulting medical professionals.

6. Coordination and Balance Deteriorate

To stay balanced, the vestibular (inner ear), proprioceptive (body position), and ocular systems cooperate. These mechanisms become less effective with age, which causes problems with balance and coordination. For instance, the elderly often struggles to maintain stability due to the vestibular system, which provides information about head position and motion, declining in function.

Additionally, as people age, their proprioception—the body's awareness of its position in space—decreases. Walking on uneven ground, climbing stairs, and simply maintaining balance while standing can be challenging for people with poor proprioception. Seniors may be more prone to trip or lose their balance if their ability to sense their body's location is compromised.

7. Health Issues and Long-Term Illness

The risk of falls is greatly increased by chronic conditions such as diabetes, Parkinson's disease, cardiovascular disease, and arthritis. Joint stiffness and discomfort from arthritis make mobility more challenging. Peripheral neuropathy, a condition in which the nerves in the legs and feet become devoid of feeling, can be brought on by diabetes. This can increase the risk of falling by making it harder to feel the floor and precisely identify movement.

Walking difficulties and tremors might be symptoms of Parkinson's disease, a disorder that affects movement and coordination. Dizziness or weakness can be a symptom of cardiovascular problems that affect the heart and circulation, particularly when standing or exercising. Because chronic illnesses can influence physical function and interact with one another in different ways, seniors who have them are often at a higher risk.

8. Reduced Reaction Time and Cognitive Deterioration

Cognitive alterations like dementia or mild cognitive impairment (MCI) might make it more difficult for a person to evaluate situations accurately and react quickly. It might be challenging for seniors to recover from slips or unexpected movements because they may have poor decision-making skills or shorter reaction times. The danger of falling is increased when people with memory difficulties neglect to use mobility aids like walkers or canes.

Confusion or disorientation can also result from cognitive disability, especially in strange situations. Due to their inability to properly anticipate or navigate environmental hazards, seniors with these impairments may be at an increased risk of falling.

9. Home Configuration and Environmental Risks

Falls are frequently caused by environmental hazards in the home, such as crowded flooring, loose carpets, and inadequate illumination. Kitchens and bathrooms are particularly hazardous due to their slick flooring. Non-slip mats, handrails in restrooms, and adequate lighting in corridors and stairwells are examples of essential features that may be absent from homes that are not built with senior safety in mind.

Elderly people who live alone are in significantly higher danger since they cannot have assistance getting around their houses safely. Changing the environment, removing hazards, and making sure assistive devices are accessible and used when needed are all part of fall prevention.

Seniors deal with several interrelated fall-related issues. A complex network of risk factors is created by declines in muscle strength, flexibility, vision, and balance as well as medical conditions, medications, cognitive decline, and environmental hazards. On the other hand, by changing their lifestyle, becoming more aware, and performing specific balancing exercises, seniors can increase their strength, stability, and confidence. The good news is that a lot of fall prevention strategies, like improving balance and strength and altering the surroundings, are very successful in reducing the risk of falls and improving quality of life.

How Improving Balance Can Improve Stability, Posture, And Self-Assurance

For seniors, balance is essential because it greatly affects their posture, confidence, and general stability, all of which enhance their quality of life. As they age, many seniors lose their balance, which impairs their physical stability and their capacity to carry out everyday tasks safely and independently. In addition to lowering the risk of falls, improving one's sense of balance has major psychological and physical benefits. Take a closer look at how improved balance improves stability, posture, and confidence.

1. Gaining Self-Belief through Improved Equilibrium

Due to their decreased balance, many seniors feel anxious and uneasy, especially when it comes to mobility and the risk of falling. Their quality of life may eventually suffer as a result of this fear, which may lead to limited mobility or avoidance of certain activities. Seniors who engage in activities that improve their balance might recover control over their movements and grow more confident in their physical capabilities.

- Increasing Self-Sufficiency in Physical Activities: Elderly people with better balance are more independent and may walk about more easily without needing assistance from others. A stable, controlled balance makes it easier and more manageable to walk, climb stairs, and even perform everyday household tasks. A strong sense of independence is fostered by this increased freedom, which also increases self-confidence and promotes an active lifestyle.

- Reducing Anxiety Associated with Falls: One of the most prevalent worries among seniors is the fear of falling, which often results in a cycle of inactivity that further impairs strength and balance. Regular balancing exercises help seniors become more resilient and reduce their fear of falling. Exercises for balance educate the body to react quickly and adjust to uneven surfaces or abrupt changes in motion, which can reduce the risk of falls and foster a sense of security. Given that elders feel more safe in their everyday activities and routines, this psychological benefit may be equally as important as the physical ones.

- Promote Social Interaction: Increased social engagement may also follow from better stability and balance. Seniors who feel good about their physical capabilities are more likely to participate in social events, family reunions, and group activities. Social interaction fosters an environment that supports an active, involved lifestyle and is crucial for mental health. Therefore, having confidence in one's ability to balance extends beyond physical movements to enhance social well-being and combat feelings of loneliness or isolation that are common among seniors.

2. Enhancing Posture with Balance Exercise

Maintaining proper body alignment reduces the strain on muscles, ligaments, and joints, and this requires good posture. Elderly people frequently have poor posture because of weakened muscles, reduced mobility, and ingrained behaviors. By strengthening the core muscles, bringing the spine into alignment, and promoting an upright posture, balance exercise naturally improves posture.

- Building Up Your Core Muscles: Both posture and balance depend on having a strong core. Seniors who perform balancing exercises engage the lower back and abdominal muscles, which are core muscles that support the spine. The maintenance of an upright posture depends on these muscles. Strong core muscles make it easier to sit or stand up straight, reduce lower back pain, and stop slouching. Standing on one leg or doing controlled weight shifts are examples of balance training exercises that are especially helpful in building core strength and improving posture.

- Reducing Muscle Tension and Adjusting the Spine: Seniors who perform balance exercises can properly align their spine, which eases the strain on their neck and back muscles. Weight is evenly distributed when the spine is in alignment, which lessens the pressure on any one group of muscles or joints. Exercises for balance that incorporate attentive alignment, like heel-to-toe walking or tandem stance (one foot in front of the other), assist the body in maintaining a straight spine while keeping the chest open and the shoulders back. Repeating these exercises over time will help to improve bad posture, ease tense muscles, and improve the comfort of standing and sitting for long periods.

- Promoting the Health of Joints: Joint health is significantly impacted by posture, especially in the hips, knees, and ankles. Often brought on by weak muscles or poor balance, bad posture can lead to misaligned joints and more strain on the ligaments and cartilage. By promoting proper alignment, balance exercises improve joint stability and reduce the risk of joint deterioration. Improved joint health allows seniors to engage in daily activities with a lower risk of pain or injury, encouraging a mobile lifestyle.

3. Increasing Stability in Everyday Tasks

Avoiding falls and maintaining control over one's movements require stability, especially while negotiating uneven terrain, changing directions, or managing quick weight shifts. Improved stability for elders refers to the capacity to carry out daily tasks with confidence and ease. Tasks requiring strong, coordinated muscles and good footing include walking, bending, reaching, and lifting objects.

- Building Up the Muscles Needed for Stability: Stability requires stronger legs and hips, which can be achieved by lower-body workouts like squats, heel-to-toe walking, and leg lifts. Seniors who train these muscles gain greater motor control and are less prone to trip or make mistakes. For everyday tasks requiring extended weight bearing, such as climbing stairs or carrying groceries, lower-body stability is especially crucial. More stable seniors are less prone to sustain joint problems or fall suddenly while going about their daily activities.

- Enhancing Reaction Time and Coordination: Balance training exercises including weight shifting, step-ups, and standing marches enhance stability while also enhancing coordination and reaction time. Rapid and accurate reactions are necessary when handling unforeseen movement changes, such as an abrupt slope or barrier. Because the body is better able to steady itself during sudden changes, a faster reaction time reduces the chance of losing balance and falling. Seniors who are coordinated and stable feel more secure going about their daily lives, which motivates them to stay active and involved in a range of circumstances.

- Promoting Fluidity in Movement and Gait: As seniors' balance improves, so does their stride, or style of walking. Exercises for balance reduce the chance of stumbling or dragging the feet by promoting smoother, more controlled steps. Exercises that enhance stride and foot placement, such as tandem stance and heel-to-toe walking, make every step more deliberate. Maintaining confidence and lowering the chance of falling are made possible by a steady stride, which also helps to maintain an even speed and increases physical endurance.

- Facilitating Mobility That Is Safer and More Confident: Finally, stability allows older people to move about safely. In addition to walking, stable footing facilitates climbing stairs, getting in and out of cars, and standing up from a seated position. A strong base makes it easier to move around safely, confidently, and actively engage with one's environment. Stable seniors can walk with purpose and exhibit less hesitancy when reaching for high shelves or moving through busy areas.

Improving balance in older adults has several advantages beyond just improving physical health. A stronger foundation for independent living, mobility, and a better quality of life is formed by improved posture, stability, and confidence. In addition to preventing falls and accidents, seniors who improve their balance also encourage a self-assured and physically fit lifestyle. By encouraging social interaction and self-reliance while reducing anxiety and dread related to mobility, balance exercises might result in mental empowerment. To put it briefly, balancing training is a ground-breaking method that greatly enhances seniors' everyday lives and sustains their mental and physical well-being for many years.

CHAPTER 2: GETTING READY FOR BALANCE ACTIVITIES

Safety Advice And Things To Think About

As we age, maintaining and improving our balance becomes crucial for our health since it reduces the chance of falls, boosts mobility, and encourages independence. To prevent harm, engaging in any kind of physical activity—especially balance exercises—requires the utmost caution. Seniors who perform balance exercises should take into account the following crucial safety precautions:

1. Speak with a Medical Expert

Consult a healthcare professional before starting any fitness program, particularly if you have a history of a sedentary lifestyle or preexisting health issues. Your physical therapist or doctor can:

- Consider your physical limitations and current state of health.
- Give specific exercise recommendations based on your demands and any possible risks.

- Advise on exercises to avoid based on any mobility or balance problems.

This initial action lays a strong basis for your fitness quest.

2. Decide on a Suitable Degree of Activity

Senior fitness levels vary greatly, so pick exercises that suit your degree of competence. You will gradually build strength and confidence if you begin with beginner-level exercises, especially if you're new to balancing routines. Advanced exercises should not be rushed into because this increases the risk of injury and falls. Your body can safely adjust if you start with easy activities and work your way up to more complex ones.

You can personalize a variety of balancing exercises. For instance, to improve balance before trying a single-leg stand on your own, start by clinging to a sturdy object, such as the back of a chair.

3. Make Use of Assistance When Required

An additional layer of security is offered by using a sturdy object for support, like a wall, countertop, or chair. When performing exercises like heel-to-toe walking and single-leg stands, support aids in maintaining your equilibrium. You may start to rely less on assistance as you get more at ease. Make sure the support you're using is stable at all times. A wall should be clear of any decorations or potentially dangerous items, and a chair should have a non-slip base.

4. Make Room

A secure training space is essential. Make sure your training area is clear of any obstructions that could cause you to trip or slip before you start, such as loose cables, clutter, or rugs. You can move around without worrying about running into furniture or slipping on something little when you have enough room. A well-lit area makes it easier to see what you're doing and reduces the chance of tripping. To increase stability and grip, install a yoga mat or exercise mat in your designated training area, or choose non-slip flooring.

5. Dress Comfortably and Wear Appropriate Footwear

When performing balancing exercises, use supportive, non-slip shoes. Shoes with a firm grip and a snug fit provide a stable foundation for standing activities and help prevent slips. It is not advised to wear socks on tiled or wooden floors unless you are using a non-slip pad.

Dress comfortably in loose-fitting clothing that doesn't restrict your range of motion. Choose clothes that let you move freely in all directions rather than ones with long hems that could trip you up.

6. Before Working Out, Warm up

By promoting blood flow to vital areas and relaxing muscles and joints, a proper warm-up gets your body ready for exercise. Because it reduces the risk of strain or damage during the main activity, this stage is especially important for seniors.

Balance exercises should be warmed up with the following:

- The ankles can be released with the aid of ankle rolls.
- To strengthen your leg muscles, march slowly in place.
- Upper body stress is relieved with shoulder and neck rolls.

Balance exercises are safer and more efficient when you warm up for five to ten minutes. This increases flexibility and gets your muscles ready for more challenging tasks.

7. Focus on Form Rather than Speed

Instead of rushing through the balance exercises, concentrate on keeping proper technique. An increased risk of falling might result from poor form, which can strain muscles and joints. You may gradually activate the right muscles and develop stability by moving slowly and deliberately.

For instance, instead of trying to raise your leg too high or balance for too long during a single-leg stand, focus on keeping your spine straight and your core active. Your ability and endurance will gradually increase with time as long as you use good form.

8. Engage in Conscious Breathing

Although breathing may not seem to have anything to do with balance exercises, it is crucial for controlling movement and maintaining composure, especially during challenging activities. Tension is released by deep, focused breathing, which gives you more control over your body.

For instance, taking calm, deep breaths may help you relax and steady your movements during a balancing exercise where you might feel unpleasant. Combining movement and breathing enhances concentration and makes it easier to stay balanced when performing challenging tasks.

9. Pay Attention to Your Body and Take Breaks as Necessary

Following your body's cues is one of the most important safety precautions. Stop and take a break if you experience any pain, dizziness, or discomfort during an exercise session. It's better to rest and adjust than to put yourself in danger because pushing through discomfort could lead to injury.

Muscle fatigue during balance exercises is normal because it can be physically taxing. On the other hand, severe pain or a feeling of unsteadiness suggests that you should modify your exercise or rest schedule. Before proceeding, consult your physician or physical therapist if the discomfort continues.

10. Drink Enough Water

Although it might seem like a minor issue, staying hydrated is essential for healthy activities. Dizziness, fatigue, and even muscle cramps brought on by dehydration raise the risk of falling and getting hurt while performing balancing exercises.

Throughout your workout, have a water bottle close at hand and take a sip as needed. Avoid consuming large quantities of water at once as this could make you feel bloated or uneasy when working out. Maintaining proper hydration will help you stay focused and energetic so you can maximize each practice while being safe.

11. Make Small, Steady Progress

Pace yourself because improving balance takes time. Workout duration, intricacy, or difficulty should be gradually increased until you feel prepared. If you're comfortable with basic exercises, for instance, you could move on to more challenging intermediate ones, including performing movements on your own.

Avoid setting unattainable objectives or exerting yourself excessively, as they can result in discontent or, worse, harm. It takes time to achieve equilibrium, and small, gradual changes over time are safer and more effective.

12. After Working Out, Relax

A cool-down routine after your balancing exercises helps to release tension, improve flexibility, and relax your muscles. Stretching gently can assist release tension from the workout, especially in the shoulders, back, and legs.

- To ease leg strain, a simple cool-down could include calf and hamstring movements.
- Stretches for the neck and shoulders assist release of tension in the upper body.
- Using deep breathing techniques might help you relax and reduce your pulse rate.

Your balancing exercises might be safer and more enjoyable if you take these safety measures and concerns into account. Gaining strength, stability, and confidence can be achieved by paying attention to your body, staying aware of your emotions, and moving at your own pace. When it comes to gradually increasing your mobility and balance, keep in mind that safety and consistency go hand in hand.

Space Preparation And Necessary Equipment

For balance exercises, especially for seniors, it is essential to create a welcoming and safe environment. Having the right equipment and organizing your workspace can greatly enhance your workout results and lower your risk of injury.

Picking the Proper Location

Selecting a suitable setting is the first step in getting ready for balancing exercises. When choosing the ideal location, keep the following points in mind:

1. Flat, Non-Slip Surface: To prevent tripping and slipping hazards, choose a location with a firm, level surface. Exercise mats and carpets are beneficial because they provide more padding and traction.

2. Proper Lighting: A well-lit area is essential for maintaining equilibrium since it allows for excellent vision. Clear visibility of the surroundings is ensured by sufficient artificial light in the evening and natural light during the day.

3. Enough Room: Ensure that there is adequate room to go about without running into walls or furniture. Exercises

involving arm or leg motions for balance should be done in a space that is at least five feet by five feet to prevent feeling confined.

4. Accessible Support: It's important to have help close by, especially for newcomers. This may be a stable chair, wall, or countertop that you could cling to in case you need to. Verify that the support is sturdy and at a reachable height.

Necessary Tools for Exercises Involving Balance

Even while many balancing exercises may be done with minimal equipment, a few simple tools can make a big difference and provide stability and safety.

1. For both standing and sitting, a chair with a sturdy, non-slip base is perfect. It enables safe mobility and offers a strong platform for support. Select a chair with a backrest and no wheels for maximum stability.

2. A comfortable, padded surface for standing, sitting, or kneeling is offered by yoga or exercise mats. Because it keeps you from slipping, it's particularly useful for activities that need you to stand still or go forth and backward. Mats that are thicker—between 5 and 8 mm—are more comfortable and stable.

3. By adding a small amount of resistance to a range of balancing activities, resistance bands are an excellent way to strengthen the arms, legs, and core. With the range of resistance levels available in these bands, seniors can begin with less resistance and progress to medium or heavy resistance as their strength increases. For safe use, bands must be securely fastened or held in place.

4. A foam cushion or balancing pad is a slightly unstable surface that encourages the body to use its stabilizing muscles, which improves balance and coordination. Seniors can improve their stability in dynamic environments by using balance pads or foam cushions, which offer a little challenge to their workouts. To practice securely when you first start, position the pad close to a sturdy support.

5. Adding a small amount of resistance, light hand weights or ankle weights can enhance strength-building exercises. These are optional but beneficial for strengthening the core and lower body, which improves balance. Start with weights between one and three pounds, emphasizing proper form and control.

6. Stability balls can be used to assess balance and activate the core for more experienced users. Although caution is

advised to prevent instability, they are suitable for both seated and some standing exercises. Use the ball in a clear space with adjacent assistance to be safe.

Setting Up the Area

A few adjustments might make the space even more welcoming and suitable for balancing exercises after the room and equipment have been selected. Take into account the following preparation advice to guarantee safety:

1. Get rid of any possible obstacles that could impede mobility or lead to tripping, like tables, cords, or rugs. An open space encourages unrestricted movement and reduces the risk of unintentional falls.

2. Mark starting points or reference lines on the floor with painter's tape for workouts that call for exact foot placements. Accuracy is improved and steady positioning is maintained.

3. The ideal temperature for balance exercises is a pleasant, moderate one. A little warmer environment—not too hot, though—can help muscles maintain their suppleness. Avoid drafts because they can cause chills or be distracting.

4. You might be able to relax and concentrate better with light background music. Select calming music or noises that don't disrupt your breathing or movement rhythm.

5. It's critical to stay hydrated during any activity. Easy breaks are made possible by having water around, especially during prolonged workouts.

Rules for the Use and Upkeep of Equipment

For both performance and safety, equipment must be used and maintained properly. Here are some tips for maintaining equipment:

1. Check for Wear and Tear: Examine all equipment for wear or damage before each use, paying special attention to balance pads and resistance bands. For instance, a ripped resistance band could break and cause injury.

2. Equipment should be stabilized and secured. Make sure the chair, balance pad, and stability ball are all firmly in place before you start working out. During a movement, unstable equipment may move, making a fall more likely.

3. Safe Equipment Storage: To prevent cluttering the workout area or posing a trip hazard, keep all exercise equipment in

one designated location. To keep the environment tidy, keep the equipment organized in a nearby basket or storage bin.

4. Equipment should be cleaned frequently. Over time, dust and perspiration can accumulate on weights, mats, and other surfaces. To guarantee cleanliness and traction, clean the equipment after every session. Make use of mild cleaning agents that won't harm the textiles.

Having the right tools and a tidy workspace is essential when getting ready for balancing exercises. The foundation for safe and effective balancing training is a well-lit, open, and secure area. Essential pieces of equipment that offer the necessary support include a sturdy chair, exercise mat, and balance pad; resistance bands and small weights further enhance the benefits.

By creating a secure, comfortable, and orderly environment, seniors can maximize their experience with balance exercises and confidently concentrate on each task. Maintaining and setting up the equipment properly can make every session enjoyable, fulfilling, and—above all—safe.

CHAPTER 3: BREATHING METHODS TO PROMOTE STABILITY AND BALANCE

Overview Of Breathing For Equilibrium

Breathing is a vital but sometimes overlooked aspect of physical health, especially when it comes to enhancing coordination, balance, and stability. Everyone breathes, so it might seem straightforward, yet how we breathe can have a big effect on our bodies and minds. Mindful breathing becomes an essential part of a senior's wellness toolkit if they want to improve their balance and prevent falls. We can improve core stability, relax the mind, and strengthen the body's natural reactions to changes in position and movement by concentrating on breathing exercises that support balance.

The ability to control one's bodily position, whether it is moving or not, is the basic definition of balance. Your neural system, muscles, and bones must all function in harmony to maintain your stability in order to achieve proper balance. Deep, intentional breathing can help synchronize these systems, enabling more control and coordination when moving.

By engaging the core muscles, the body's main stabilizer, breathing has an impact on balance. The diaphragm, transverse abdominis, and pelvic floor muscles are among the core muscles that are essential for keeping one's posture straight and avoiding falls. These muscles are slightly affected by each inhalation and exhalation, which can either increase stability or lead to instability if breathing is pushed or shallow. Balance depends on both the mind-body connection and the foundation of the body, both of which are enhanced by controlled breathing.

Maintaining balance involves more than simply physical exertion; it also calls for mental concentration. The parasympathetic nervous system also referred to as the "rest and digest" system, is triggered by mindful breathing and aids in mental relaxation and anxiety reduction. This relaxation response is particularly crucial for seniors because it reduces stress, which throws off balance by creating unnecessary tension in the body. The body can focus more effectively on preserving stability and react swiftly to positional changes without losing equilibrium when the mind is at ease. By putting the body in a relaxed yet alert state, mindful breathing gets it ready for balance exercises.

One of the most important muscles for breathing and balance is the diaphragm, a dome-shaped muscle located behind the lungs. The diaphragm contracts and descends during deep, full breaths, enabling the lungs to expand and fill with air. In addition to improving oxygen delivery to the body, this exercise strengthens and stabilizes the core. Conversely, shallow or chest-centered breathing weakens the core and impairs overall balance by decreasing diaphragm participation.

By working with other core muscles to generate stability, a strong, flexible diaphragm provides a strong basis for balance. By concentrating on diaphragmatic breathing, also referred to as "belly breathing," we can engage the core and prime it to react to workouts involving balance or posture adjustments. With repeated practice, this type of breathing strengthens the core overall and enhances balance and muscle control.

The body's capacity to adapt to sudden movements or changes in the terrain usually determines balance. The body's natural reaction to a stumble is to catch itself, which necessitates rapid muscle reaction and coordination. Movement-based breathing exercises can improve reflexes and reaction time by teaching the body to respond quickly and calmly. Breathing is linked with movements that improve balance and body control in daily situations, making it more than just a lonely activity.

Proprioception, or the awareness of one's body's position in space, is also enhanced by deliberate breathing. Proprioception enables the body to make automatic adjustments to prevent falls since it quickly recognizes changes in posture. In addition to strengthening your core and promoting mental relaxation, focused breathing exercises enhance your brain's perception of and response to physical movements, which enhances your overall balance.

Although it might seem like a small exercise, mindful breathing offers a strong foundation for both mental and physical health. Seniors who use breathing exercises to improve their balance typically report feeling safer and more assured when moving around in daily life. Controlled breathing reduces the risk of falling because it strengthens the core, relaxes the mind, and improves body awareness.

Whether used alone or in conjunction with a balancing exercise, intentional breathing is a crucial strategy for preserving stability and reducing the chance of falling. By starting with these breathing exercises, seniors can develop resilience, maintain a connection to their bodies, and benefit from confident, healthful movement for many years to come.

Diaphragmatic Breathing (belly)

The diaphragm, a dome-shaped muscle situated above the abdomen and beneath the lungs, is used in the diaphragmatic breathing technique, often known as belly breathing. This method offers a straightforward but efficient way to boost oxygen flow, calm the nervous system, and engage the balance-related core muscles. For seniors, diaphragmatic breathing is a gentle and efficient method of increasing stability and coordination, as well as body awareness and core engagement.

In order to achieve deep, controlled breaths, diaphragmatic breathing aims to fully engage the diaphragm. Diaphragmatic breathing concentrates on the lower lungs, expanding the belly as you inhale and contracting it as you exhale, in contrast to shallow breathing, which primarily uses the chest muscles. This deeper breath promotes calmness, stability, and a natural activation of the core.

Benefits of Diaphragmatic Breathing for Equilibrium

1. By strengthening the diaphragm and core muscles, deep breathing creates the solid base of support needed for good posture and balance. The diaphragm and core muscles, especially the transverse abdominis, cooperate as you

breathe deeply, keeping you stable in a range of circumstances.

2. By focusing on your body, diaphragmatic breathing fosters mindfulness and a better sense of your location in space. Proprioception, or increased body awareness, is crucial for balance because it enables you to react quickly to changes in your surroundings or position.

3. The parasympathetic nervous system is triggered by deep belly breathing, which reduces tension and encourages relaxation. Elderly people benefit most from mental relaxation since it reduces stress and balances the body's reactions to activity.

4. The best possible oxygen intake is made possible by diaphragmatic breathing, which increases physical endurance, energy, and focus—all of which are critical for preserving balance and coordination when moving.

Methods for Diaphragmatic Breathing Practice

This is a detailed guide on how to practice diaphragmatic breathing:

1. You can either comfortably lie down or sit in a chair with your feet resting on the floor. Two hands should be placed on your chest and abdomen, respectively.

2. Breathe in slowly via your nose, letting the diaphragm expand and your stomach rise. While the hand on your chest remains largely motionless, feel the one on your abdomen moves outward. Make an effort to breathe in your lower lungs.

3. Exhale slowly through your lips, letting the diaphragm relax and your abdomen return to your spine. While the hand on your chest stays steady, the one on your abdomen should drop.

4. For five to ten breaths, repeat this while maintaining a steady, calm rhythm. Aim for several seconds between each inhalation and exhalation. Try to keep your breathing controlled and fluid.

After you've perfected the technique, think about integrating diaphragmatic breathing into routine tasks like walking, stair climbing, or balancing training. With time, this breathing pattern will become more instinctive, enabling you to stay focused, steady, and grounded while performing your everyday tasks.

Box Breathing For Concentration And Calm

Box breathing, sometimes referred to as four-square breathing, is a straightforward but incredibly effective method for controlling your breathing, enhancing focus, and calming your mind. Seniors who wish to improve their stability and balance while also lowering their stress and anxiety levels can benefit from this methodical breathing technique. You can attain a state of calm that enhances your general well-being and gets your body ready for exercise by engaging in box breathing exercises.

During inbox breathing, you take a breath, hold it for four counts, then release it. This method creates a rhythmic breathing pattern that promotes calmness and mental clarity. The "box" stands for the breathing cycle's four equal sides, which encourages control and balance.

Benefits of Box Breathing for Concentration and Balance

1. By inducing the relaxation response, box breathing lowers stress hormones and promotes feelings of calm. Elderly people who experience less stress may have better balance because tension can occasionally lead to instability and a fear of falling.

2. Box breathing's methodical approach helps people focus and concentrate better. This clarity is particularly helpful before engaging in physical activities that require mental acuity, such as balance exercises.

3. Because box breathing concentrates on the breath, it encourages mindfulness and a greater awareness of your body. Because it makes it easier to understand your physical presence in space, this enhanced body awareness is essential for balance.

4. Box breathing's gradual, controlled breathing pattern optimizes oxygen intake, which is essential for vitality and athletic performance. Greater balance is the outcome of improved muscle function and coordination brought about by increased oxygen flow.

5. Box breathing encourages relaxation by assisting in heart rate regulation. When performing balance exercises, a constant heart rate enables more regulated movements, which enhances physical performance.

Methods for Box Breathing Practice

This is a detailed guide on box breathing:

1. Locate a peaceful area where you may easily sit or lie down, or sit in a chair with your feet flat on the floor. Close your eyes and unwind for a while if it makes you feel more at ease.

2. Feel the air filling your lungs as you take a slow, four-count breath through your nose. Extend your abdomen as you inhale.

3. For four counts, hold your breath. Keep your posture relaxed and let go of any stress in your body at this time.

4. For four counts, slowly expel the air through your mouth, letting your abdomen fall as you do so. As you breathe, picture tension and stress leaving your body.

5. Before you take the next breath, hold your breath for four more counts. Keep your posture relaxed and savor the peace of the moment.

6. Maintain a four-count beat and pay attention to your breathing as you repeat this cycle for five to ten minutes.

Gently bring your focus back to your breathing if your thoughts start to stray.

Simply said, box breathing is a part of everyday routines. To calm your mind and get your body ready, you can do it before doing balancing exercises. It can also help you regain focus and balance during stressful or anxious moments of the day.

For instance, spend a few minutes practicing box breathing if you're experiencing anxiety or being overwhelmed. You may be able to ground yourself and deal with issues more composedly and lucidly if you follow this easy exercise.

Additionally, incorporating box breathing into your warm-up routine before any physical activity will enhance readiness and focus. Box breathing for a few minutes can help your body and mind get ready for the workouts ahead, keeping you focused and in the moment.

Box breathing is a useful technique with numerous advantages for mental and physical well-being. For seniors who want to increase their stability and balance, this structured breathing method enhances focus, encourages relaxation, and fortifies the mind-body link. You can cultivate a sense of calm that enhances your physical activity and overall quality of life by incorporating box breathing into your daily practice. Whether used as a stress-reduction technique or before balance exercises, box breathing is an essential technique that promotes long-term stability and resilience.

Coordination Of Breath And Movement

The idea of breath coordination with movement is crucial for enhancing physical performance, particularly for elderly people looking to increase their stability and balance. This method focuses on aligning your breathing with your movements, creating a natural rhythm that encourages both physical activity and mental and physical focus. Gaining knowledge of and expertise with breath coordination will enhance your workout experience overall and provide you greater control over your body when performing balancing exercises.

The Importance of Coordinating Breath

There are several reasons why breath synchrony is crucial.

1. Enhances Stability: Breathing and movement coordination can provide a strong basis for physical activities. Engaging your core muscles during inhalation and exhalation aids in maintaining balance and posture, which facilitates easier transitions between activities.

2. Boosts Oxygen Flow: You can make sure that your muscles get a constant supply of oxygen by coordinating your breathing with your movements. Because it encourages muscular function and endurance, this increased oxygen

supply is essential for optimal performance, particularly during physical exercise.

3. Enhances Mind-Body Connection: By combining movement with breathing, you may increase your awareness of your body's alignment and posture while working out. Better body mechanics may result from this heightened awareness, which is particularly beneficial for elderly people who wish to increase their balance and prevent falls.

4. You can better control your pulse rate and keep a steady pace when you can control your breathing while you're moving. This control maintains you within a safe and comfortable range and aids in the management of physical exertion.

5. Facilitates Focus and Relaxation: Throughout the action, breath synchronization fosters a calmer mental state. You can focus on your form and motions by focusing on your breathing to assist you get rid of distractions and anxiousness.

How to Work on Movement and Breath Coordination

For seniors in particular, here is a detailed guide on how to practice breath coordination with movement:

1. Select a basic exercise or activity, such as modest arm raises, standing marches, or sitting leg lifts. Verify if the movement is within your capabilities and comfort zone.

2. Take some time to connect with your breath before starting the movement. Breathe diaphragmatically for a few cycles to focus yourself and get ready for the workout.

3. Choose a breathing technique that goes well with the movement. For instance:
   - As you raise your arms or legs in preparation for the activity, take a breath.
   - As you complete the movement, such as raising your arm or leg, slowly release your breath. This aids in in-body stabilization and core activation.
   - Return to the starting posture by taking another breath while lowering your arm or leg slowly.

4. Focus on maintaining a steady rhythm between your breathing and movement while you practice. Try to make

the transition smooth and easy while remaining deliberate
and in control of your activities.

5. Throughout the exercise, pay attention to your breathing and
   body. Bring your focus back on the synchronization of your
   breathing and movements if your thoughts stray. This
   methodical technique might enhance your overall efficacy and
   experience.

Examples of Exercises for Breathing Coordination

*Activities that can improve breath coordination include the
following:*

1. Arm lifts while seated:
- Lift both arms in the air and take a breath.
- Lower your arms back down and exhale.

2. Marches while standing:
- As you bring one knee up to hip level, take a breath.
- Exhale as you alternate legs and bring the knee back to
  the floor.

3. Lifting your legs:

- Raise one leg to the side and take a breath.
- As you bring the leg back to its initial position, release your breath.

4. Soft twists:

- Take a breath and then twist your torso.
- Exhale, then twist slowly to one side while maintaining stability with your core.

Breath coordination is useful in everyday life and is not just for scheduled exercise. For instance:

- Take a few breaths in, then let them out. This can help you walk with better posture and maintain a steady pace.
- Managing your breath while sweeping or gardening is one example of a household task. As you are ready to rise or reach, take a breath, and as you do so, release it.
- To increase focus and relaxation, integrate breath coordination into your yoga or stretching routine by linking your breath to each pose or stretch.

An efficient method for enhancing your stability, balance, and overall physical performance is to coordinate your breathing with your movements. In addition to improving your physical capabilities, synchronizing your breathing with your movements strengthens the bond between your mind and body. Because it promotes a more mindful approach to physical exercise, promoting calm and focus while reducing the risk of falling, this practice is particularly beneficial for older adults. Including breath coordination in your everyday activities and workout routine can help you become more resilient and stable, which will enhance your quality of life in general.

Guided Relaxation For Recuperation After Physical Activity

A key component of post-exercise recovery is guided relaxation, particularly for seniors who wish to enhance their general well-being while preserving stability and balance. This method uses a series of calming suggestions to help the body and mind relax, which promotes mental clarity and physical recovery after exercise. You may enhance the benefits of your exercises and improve your sense of peace by incorporating guided relaxation into your routine.

The significance of recuperating after exercise

1. Physical Recovery: Your muscles need time to recover after physical activity. Relaxation methods can promote circulation, alleviate tense muscles, and hasten the healing process.

2. Reduction of Tension: Guided relaxation can assist reduce the physical tension that exercise might create in the body. This can result in a calmer state and lower cortisol levels.

3. Mental Clarity: Engaging in physical exercise and guided relaxation enhances mental clarity, enabling a more

focused and in-the-moment attitude. Seniors who wish to enhance their overall mental health and cognitive function will find this to be extremely beneficial.

4. For seniors who wish to maintain their range of motion, relaxation techniques can improve flexibility by promoting mild stretching and releasing tense muscles.

5. Emotional Well-Being: Following physical activity, guided relaxation can lessen the chance of anxiety or depression by fostering emotional stability and resilience.

How to Perform Guided Relaxation to Help Recuperate After Exercise

The following is a detailed guide to guided relaxation after working out:

1. Find a peaceful spot where you may sit or lie down without being disturbed. Turn down the lights, play some relaxing music, or take in the sounds of nature if you'd like.

2. Choose a comfortable position to sit or lie in. You can use your bed, a comfortable chair, or a yoga mat. Shut your eyes and take a few deep breaths to discover your core.

3. Pay attention to your breath for a time. Exhale slowly through your mouth after taking a big breath through your nose that causes your abdomen to rise. Continue doing this until your body starts to relax.

4. Work your way up your body, starting at the tips of your toes. Spend a few seconds tensing each muscle group, then relax and allow the tension to subside. For instance, tense your toes, hold them for a second, and then relax. Your feet should come first, followed by your calves, thighs, and head.

5. Once your body is at ease, visualize a calm setting. Picture yourself in a serene location, such as a mountain, beach, or woodland. Allow your mind to fully immerse itself in the experience by imagining the sounds, smells, and sensations of that place.

6. You can utilize a script or audio guide for relaxation if you'd like. These can offer detailed instructions and kind reminders to help you unwind even more. Seek out recordings designed especially for recuperation after exercise.

7. As you relax, keep taking deep, regular breaths. Take four breaths, hold them for four counts, and then release them

for four counts. Keep up this pace, letting your breathing take center stage.

8. Make a healing intention while you're sleeping. This might be a simple acknowledgment of the work you put into your workout or an affirmation. For example, "I respect my body and its capacity to recover" or even "I am thankful for my fortitude and tenacity."

9. At least ten to fifteen minutes should be spent in this peaceful state. Feel free to extend your practice if you have more time. The benefits will increase with the amount of time you spend unwinding.

10. Slowly bring your attention back to the present when you're ready to wrap up your session. Gently stretch your body, wiggle your fingers and toes, and open your eyes slowly. Spend some time evaluating your feelings before getting up or moving.

For post-exercise rehabilitation, guided relaxation is a useful tactic, especially for seniors who wish to maintain their stability, balance, and general well-being. You can enhance mental clarity, lessen stress, and encourage physical recovery by incorporating this practice into your routine. The advantages of guided relaxation can assist you in taking a more peaceful and well-rounded approach to your journey toward health and fitness, regardless of whether you use progressive muscle relaxation, visual imagery, or guided scripts. After working out, taking some time to relax creates the foundation for future progress and an enhanced quality of life.

CHAPTER 4: SIMPLE BALANCE WORKOUTS FOR SENIORS

Beginner Level

1. Heel raises while standing (with support)

Instructions:
1. Hold onto a chair for support as you stand behind it.
2. Come onto the balls of your feet by slowly raising your heels.
3. Controllably descend again. Do this 15–20 times.

Benefits:
- Increases walking endurance by strengthening calves.
- Improves ankle flexibility, which is important for equilibrium.

2. Heel Raises on One Leg (With Support)

Instructions:
1. Support yourself with one hand on a chair.
2. Raise the heel of the standing leg and lift one foot off the ground.

3. Lower each leg and repeat ten repetitions.

Benefits:
- Improves one-leg balance by strengthening calves.
- Decreases the chance of falls by improving ankle stability.

3. Rocking back and forth while receiving assistance

Instructions:
1. Hold a chair in your hands.
2. Rock back to your heels after shifting your weight on your toes.
3. Do this 15–20 times.

Benefits:
- Improves balance by strengthening the ankles.
- Enhances proprioception, or awareness of one's body's location.

4. Tandem Position (With Assistance)

Instructions:
1. Hold a chair while standing with one foot in front of the other.
2. Switch feet after holding for 10 to 30 seconds.

Benefits:

- Reduces the base of support, which tests equilibrium.
- Increases the stability of the lower leg muscles.

5. Narrow Position (No Assistance)

Instructions:

1. Place your hands by your sides and your feet close together.
2. Hold for 10 to 30 seconds while paying attention to your balance.

Benefits:

- Promotes improved balance by using the core muscles.
- Strengthens the legs, which helps with stability.

6. Standing with a weight shift from side to side

Instructions:

1. Hold a chair while standing with your feet hip-width apart.
2. Lift the opposing foot a little by shifting weight to one side.
3. Do 15–20 reps on alternate sides.

Benefits:

- Promotes stability by strengthening the hip and leg muscles.

- Enhances equilibrium, which is necessary for day-to-day tasks.

7. Stand on One Leg (With Support)

Instructions:
1. Hold a chair in one hand while standing behind it.
2. For ten to thirty seconds, raise one foot while maintaining balance on the other.
3. Repeat after switching legs.

Benefits:
- Increases stability and strength in the lower body.
- Promotes leg and ankle flexibility, which lowers the risk of falls.

8. Toe raises while standing (with support)

Instructions:
1. Hold a chair for balance while standing with your feet hip-width apart.
2. Keep your heels on the floor and raise your toes.
3. For 15–20 repetitions, lower and repeat.

Benefits:

- Increases lower leg muscular mass, which promotes stability.
- Strengthens the ankles, which is important for gait and balance.

9. Bending the knee slightly (with support)

Instructions:

1. Place your feet hip-width apart and stand behind a chair.
2. Maintain a straight back while holding the chair and bending your knees slightly.
3. Get back up on your feet. Repeat ten to fifteen times.

Benefits:

- Promotes joint stability by strengthening the knee and thighs.
- Increases knee suppleness, facilitating practical motions.

10. Bending Sideways While Seated

Instructions:

1. Take a tall seat in a chair with your arms at your sides and your feet flat on the ground.
2. For support, place your right hand on the chair's side.

3. Reach toward the ceiling with your left arm raised over your head.
4. Stretch the left side of your torso by bending slightly to the right. For 15 to 30 seconds, hold.
5. Go back to the middle and swap sides. For each side, repeat three times.

Benefits:
- Increases the range of motion and flexibility of the spine.
- Bolsters the stability of the core by strengthening the oblique muscles.

11. Weight Shift While Seated (Side-to-Side)

Instructions:
1. Place your hands on your lap and sit upright with your feet hip-width apart.
2. Raise your left hip a little off the chair by shifting your weight to your right hip.
3. Return to the center after holding for a short while.
4. Repeat after moving to the left. Do ten to fifteen shifts on each side.

Benefits:
- Improves core stability, which is crucial for equilibrium.
- Increases hip strength, which lowers the chance of falls.

12. Pelvic tilt while seated forward and backward

Instructions:
1. Place your feet hip-width apart and sit on the edge of a chair.
2. Arch your lower back slightly and tilt your pelvis forward.
3. Next, round your lower back by tilting it back.
4. Repeat ten to fifteen times, carefully and slowly.

Benefits:
- Reduces lower back stress by increasing pelvic flexibility.
- Improves posture by strengthening the lower back and core muscles.

13. March 1

Instructions:
1. Take a tall stance and place your feet flat on the ground.
2. Raise and then lower your right knee toward your chest.
3. Continue for 30 to 60 seconds, switching to the left knee.

Benefits:
- Improves mobility by strengthening the hip flexors.
- Strengthens the core, improving balance and stability.

14. Forward-Seated Get to

Instructions:
1. Place your arms on your thighs and sit with your feet flat on the floor.
2. Bend forward and extend your hands to the ground.
3. Return to sitting upright after holding for a little while. Do this ten times.

Benefits:
- Increases spinal mobility by strengthening the back muscles.
- Improves stability and balance by strengthening the core.

15. Rotation of the Seated Body

Instructions:
1. Hold the chair's sides while sitting with your feet flat.
2. While maintaining a steady hip position, rotate your torso to one side.
3. Switch sides after a brief hold and a return to the center. Do this ten times.

Benefits:

- Increases upper body flexibility, which is beneficial for everyday mobility.
- Improves balance by activating the core muscles.

Intermediate Level

1. Walking on Heels

Instructions:
1. Take a tall stance and balance on your heels by raising your toes.
2. Take ten to fifteen steps forward on your heels, then straighten up.

Benefits:
- Improves foot stability by strengthening the muscles in the lower legs.
- Increases bodily awareness by improving proprioception.

2. Heel-to-toe tandem Strolling

Instructions:
1. Place one foot, heel to toe, directly in front of the other.
2. Take a step forward, pressing the toes of the front foot against the heel of the back foot.
3. Take ten steps while maintaining a tight line.

Benefits:
- A tight stance improves balance.
- Improves stability by strengthening the leg muscles.

3. Reach Forward (While Maintaining a Narrow Stance)

Instructions:
1. Place your feet close to each other.
2. Lean forward a little and extend your arms in front of you.
3. Return to standing after a few seconds of holding the reach. Do this ten times.

Benefits:
- Increases core stability, which is necessary for equilibrium.
- Increases the flexibility of the spine and shoulders.

4. Marching without assistance

Instructions:
1. Take a tall stance with your arms by your sides and your feet hip-width apart.
2. lift one leg to hip height, then lift the other knee while lowering the first.
3. March in place for 30 seconds while switching knees.

Benefits:
- Improves walking stability by strengthening the hip flexors.
- Improves balance and coordination.

5. Stand to Sit (with one leg in front of you)

Instructions:
1. Place one foot slightly forward while seated in a chair.
2. Maintaining one foot in front of you, lean forward, and push yourself up to stand.
3. Return to your seat slowly. For each leg, repeat ten times.

Benefits:
- Supports everyday motions by strengthening the legs and core.
- Challenges the distribution of weight, improving balance.

6. Squat (Unsupported)

Instructions:
1. Stand with your arms out in front of you and your feet hip-width apart.
2. Lower your hips toward the floor by bending your knees.
3. Get back to standing and do it ten to fifteen times.

Benefits:
- Promotes balance by strengthening the legs and core.
- Makes the knees and hips more flexible.

7. Stand on One Leg (With Free Leg Movement)

Instructions:
1. Raise one leg slightly while standing on the other.
2. Move the raised leg forward and backward or in tiny circles.
3. Switch legs after holding for ten to fifteen seconds.

Benefits:
- Increases joint stability and leg strength.
- Enhances balance and tests coordination.

8. Knee Bend on One Leg

Instructions:
1. Bend your knee slightly while standing on one leg.
2. Drop a couple of inches, then stand back up.
3. After ten repetitions, switch legs.

Benefits:
- Strengthens the knee and thigh muscles.
- Lowers the risk of falls by improving single-leg stability.

9. Standing to Sitting (Unsupported)

Instructions:

1. Place your feet hip-width apart and sit at the edge of a chair.
2. Without using your hands, stand up by crossing your arms over your chest.
3. Slowly take a seat again. Do this ten times.

Benefits:

- Increases lower body strength, which is necessary for movement.
- Promotes self-reliance by supporting everyday tasks.

10. Heel Raises on One Leg (With Light Support)

Instructions:

1. For light support, place your fingertips on a chair.
2. Raise the heel of the standing foot by lifting one foot.
3. Lower each leg ten times, then repeat.

Benefits:

- Increases stability and calves' strength.
- Increases ankle suppleness, promoting equilibrium.

11. Leg Raises on the Side (With Support)

Instructions:
1. Hold a chair for support as you stand next to it.
2. Without cocking your torso, raise one leg out to the side.
3. Lower each leg ten to fifteen times, then repeat.

Benefits:
- Promotes lateral stability by strengthening the hips and outer thighs.
- Increases hip suppleness, promoting equilibrium.

12. Tandem Position (No Assistance)

Instructions:
1. Place one foot in front of the other so that the heel touches the toe.
2. Switch feet after holding the position for 10 to 30 seconds.

Benefits:
- Improves stability and tests equilibrium.
- Improves mobility by strengthening the lower legs.

13. Narrow Position (With Rotation of the Neck)

Instructions:
1.   Stand with your arms relaxed and your feet close together.
2.   Rotate your head slowly back and forth.
3.   Hold, paying attention to stability, for 10 to 30 seconds.

Benefits:
- Increases leg strength and stability.
- Adds head movement, making balance more difficult.

14. Stand on One Leg (No Support)

Instructions:
1.   Raise one foot off the ground and stand erect.
2.   Switch legs after holding the position for 10 to 30 seconds.

Benefits:
- Enhances balance, which is crucial for avoiding falls.
- Increases the endurance and strength of the legs.

15. Walking on Toes

Instructions:

1. Take a tall stance and balance on your toes by lifting your heels.
2. Take ten to fifteen steps forward on your toes.

Benefits:

- Improves balance by strengthening the ankles and calves.
- Increases the flexibility of the lower legs, promoting movement.

16. Tandem Position (With Light Support and Neck Rotation)

Instructions:

1. Hold a chair lightly while standing with one foot in front of the other.
2. While maintaining your balance, turn your head from side to side.
3. Switch feet after holding for 10 to 20 seconds.

Benefits:

- Promotes balance by increasing lower body stability.
- Introduces neck movement, which tests proprioception.

Advanced Level

1. Single-Leg Stand (with Eye Movement)

Instructions:
1. Stand on one leg, with the other leg slightly raised.
2. Move your eyes side to side or up and down to test your balance.
3. Hold the position for 10-30 seconds before switching legs.

Benefits:
- Improves proprioception and balance during visual distraction.
- It strengthens the stabilizing muscles in the standing leg.

2. Tandem Toe-to-heel walking (backward)

Instructions:
1. Stand with one foot directly behind the other, heel to toe.
2. Take slow, backward steps, with the heel of the rear foot against the toes of the front.
3. Repeat for ten steps, concentrating on keeping balance.

Benefits:
- Improves lower-body muscle strength, balance, and coordination.
- Improves stability by challenging the body in an uncommon movement pattern.

3. Tandem Walking (with Neck Rotation)

Instructions:
1. Stand with one foot directly in front of the other, heel to toe.
2. Maintain your balance by slowly rotating your head to one side and then the other.
3. Walk in a straight line for about ten steps, concentrating on maintaining balance while you swivel your head.

Benefits:
- Improves balance and stability by testing coordination.
- Improves neck flexibility and proprioception, which are essential for maintaining stability.

4. Single-Legged Stand (With Arm Movement)

Instructions:

1. Stand on one leg, then lift the opposing leg off the ground.
2. Maintain your equilibrium by extending your arms to the sides or overhead.
3. Hold the position for 10-30 seconds before switching legs. Move your arms in little circles or up and down to add difficulty.

Benefits:

- Strengthens stabilizing muscles in standing legs.
- Increases balance and coordination by incorporating arm exercises.

5. Mini Lunge (Staggering Stance with Knee Bend)

Instructions:

1. Stand with one foot forward and the other back, with the rear heel lifted.
2. Bend your front knee while keeping your back leg straight, then lower your body slightly.
3. Return to the beginning position, repeating 10 times per leg.

Benefits:

- Strengthens leg muscles, including quadriceps and glutes.
- Improves balance and stability with controlled motions.

6. Walking Side by Side

Instructions:

1. Stand tall, feet hip-width apart.
2. Take a step to the right and bring your left foot to meet your right.
3. Repeat on the left side. Continue the side-to-side movement for 30 seconds.

Benefits:

- Improves lateral stability and leg strength.
- Enhances coordination and balance through dynamic movement.

7. Single Leg Knee Bend (With Light Support)

Instructions:

1. Stand on one leg, with a chair or countertop providing light support.
2. Bend the knee of the standing leg slightly to lower your torso a few inches.

3. Return to the beginning position, repeating 10 times per leg.

Benefits:
- Strengthens knee and leg muscles for better stability.
- Improves balance by emphasizing weight distribution.

8. 360-Degree

Instructions:
1. Stand with your feet hip-width apart.
2. Slowly turn your body in a full circle while glancing over each shoulder.
3. Repeat the turn 3-5 times, concentrating on balance.

Benefits:
- Enhances balance and coordination during circular movements.
- Improves stability by challenging your sense of direction.

9. Squat Hold (without Support)

Instructions:
1. Stand with your feet shoulder-width apart.
2. Lower yourself into a squat position with your knees behind your toes.

3. Squat for 10 to 30 seconds before returning to standing.

Benefits:
- Improves leg and core strength, leading to greater stability.
- Enhances endurance and balance in a functioning position.

10. Single-Leg Stand (Eyes Closed)

Instructions:
1. Stand on one leg and elevate the other foot slightly off the ground.
2. Close your eyes and keep this position for 10-30 seconds before switching legs.

Benefits:
- Improves equilibrium by reducing visual input.
- It strengthens the stabilizing muscles in the standing leg.

11. Tandem heel-to-toe walking

Instructions:
1. Stand with one foot directly in front of the other, heel to toe.
2. Walk forward with the heel of your rear foot contacting the toes of your front foot.
3. Repeat for ten steps, concentrating on keeping balance.

Benefits:
- Improves balance and coordination with a narrower stance.
- Strengthens leg muscles and increases stability.

12. Squat (without support)

Instructions:
1. Stand with your feet shoulder-width apart.
2. Squat with your back straight and chest up.
3. Return to standing and repeat for 10-15 repetitions.

Benefits:
- Increases lower body strength, which is essential for stability and mobility.
- Increases flexibility in the hips and knees.

13. Squat-to-Heel Raises (No Support)

Instructions:
1. Stand with your feet shoulder-width apart.
2. Squat and, as you rise, pull your heels off the ground.
3. Return to a standing position and do 10-15 reps.

Benefits:

- Strengthens both calves and thighs simultaneously.
- Improves coordination and stability with compound movement.

14. Single Leg Stand (with Torso Rotation)

Instructions:

1. Stand on one leg and hold a lightweight object (such as a ball) at chest level.
2. Balance on one leg and rotate your torso from side to side.
3. Hold for 10-30 seconds and then switch legs.

Benefits:

- Boosts core stability and improves balance.
- Movement tests your coordination and muscle control.

15. Standing March (with Pauses)

Instructions:

1. Stand tall, feet hip-width apart.
2. March in place, bringing your knees to hip level.
3. Pause slightly after each lift to improve balance. Continue for 30 seconds.

Benefits:
- Enhances hip flexors and improves coordination.
- Increases balance by inserting pauses.

16. Walking Backwards (with Neck Rotation)

Instructions:
1. Stand tall and take short steps backward.
2. As you walk, swivel your head and gaze over each shoulder.
3. Walk backward for roughly 10 steps while maintaining control.

Benefits:
- Improves balance and coordination.
- Strengthens lower-body muscles, particularly the hamstrings.

CHAPTER 5: ESTABLISHING A CUSTOMIZED BALANCE PROGRAM AND MONITORING RESULTS

How To Create A Weekly Calendar That Is Balanced

Creating a balanced weekly routine is essential for seniors who want to improve their overall health, particularly in terms of balance, stability, and independence. With the support of a well-thought-out plan, people may efficiently integrate exercise into their everyday lives, monitor their progress, and maintain organization. This comprehensive guide will help seniors create a well-rounded weekly program that encourages fun, safety, and physical health.

1. Evaluate Your Level of Fitness

It's important to assess your current level of fitness before starting a new regimen. This assessment will assist you in identifying your areas of strength and growth. Think about the following queries:

- How active am I at the moment? Do you now lead a sedentary lifestyle or do you often exercise?
- Do I currently have any health issues? For information on any restrictions or safety measures related to exercise, speak with your healthcare provider.
- Which hobbies are enjoyable to me? Being aware of your preferences may make it easier for you to stick to your timetable.

By taking the time to evaluate these factors, you will create a strong foundation for your habit.

2. Establish Attainable and Unambiguous Goals

Setting clear, achievable goals is the next stage after assessing your present level of fitness. These objectives will offer direction and rewards. Take into account the following SMART criteria while creating goals:

- Specific: Specify your objective (e.g., "I want to improve my balance").
- Measurable: Establish a plan for monitoring your development (e.g., "I will practice standing on one leg for 30 seconds").
- Achievable: Verify that your objectives are within your current range of fitness.

- Relevant: Make sure your goals are meaningful to you. For instance, "I want to be able to walk without support"
- Time-bound: Give your objectives a due date, such as "I want to finish this in three months."

"I will practice balance exercises for 30 minutes three times per week for the next month" is an example of a goal.

3. Make a Weekly Plan

Making a weekly schedule is a crucial first step in developing a healthy routine. You can include a range of exercises that focus on strength, flexibility, and balance in a well-organized routine. This is how to get ready:

Set aside specific days for every kind of exercise.
- Try to do strength training two or three days a week. Focus on exercises that will strengthen your upper body, legs, and core.
- Try doing balance exercises at least two or three times a week. You can include these workouts in your strength-training routine.
- Stretch or practice yoga at least two to three times a week to increase flexibility and reduce stiffness.

- Three to five days a week, do mild cardiovascular exercises like cycling or walking. Every week, try to get in at least 150 minutes of moderate-intensity exercise.

4. Include Variety

Change up your routine to keep motivated and prevent boredom. While keeping your workout engaging, you can use different exercises to target different muscle areas. Here are some suggestions:

- Try cycling, swimming, walking, or utilizing an elliptical machine to mix up your aerobic regimen.
- Use resistance bands, weights, or bodyweight exercises like lunges and squats to vary your strength training.
- Seek out engaging and amusing local fitness programs, such as water aerobics, tai chi, or chair yoga.

You can focus on several aspects of fitness while maintaining an engaging routine by combining different activities.

5. Pay Attention to Your Body

When creating your regimen, it's important to pay attention to your body. Observe your feelings both during and after working out. Some crucial things to think about are:

- When necessary, take a break to allow your body to heal. Take a break or alter your routine if you're feeling worn out or sore.
- If an exercise is too difficult, change it up. For instance, try a single-leg stand with help if you find it too challenging.
- To stay hydrated, especially during demanding activities, drink water before, during, and following exercise.

Being aware of your body's signals is essential to preventing injuries and enjoying your exercise.

6. Monitor Your Progress

Maintaining a balanced schedule requires that you keep track of your accomplishments. Maintaining a log of your workouts will help you stay motivated and track your progress. Here are several methods to track your development:

- Keep a Journal: Note your workouts, including your activities, the time you spent doing them, and your post-workout feelings.
- Use fitness trackers or apps: A lot of apps let you set goals, record your activities, and monitor your progress.

- Establish frequent check-ins: Arrange for weekly or monthly evaluations to ascertain how well you're accomplishing your goals. Adapt your regimen to your progress as necessary.

7. Remain Inspired

Keeping yourself motivated is essential to follow your routine. The following strategies will help you stay interested:

- Find a Workout Partner: Exercise can be more enjoyable and accountable when done with a companion.
- Enroll in a Group Class: By fostering social connection, community fitness classes can increase motivation.
- Celebrate Your Milestones: Take pride in your achievements, no matter how small. Give yourself a lovely gift or your favorite pastime as a reward.

8. Put Safety First

The primary concern should always be safety, particularly for elderly people. To create a secure exercise space, take into account the following recommendations:

- Select Safe Locations: Make sure the space is free of obstacles and dangers whether you're doing it out at home or in a gym.
- Wear the Right Shoes: Invest in traction-enhancing, supportive shoes.
- Use Support When Necessary: To ensure your safety during workouts, don't be scared to use chairs, walls, or other supports.

9. Be Adaptive and Flexible

Be ready to adjust your schedule as needed because life can be unpredictable. If you have to change your regimen or miss an activity, don't give up. Focus on getting back on course as soon as you can.

Establishing a well-rounded weekly schedule is a prudent investment in your health and welfare. By determining your level of fitness, setting reasonable goals, planning your schedule, adding variety, and putting safety first, you may develop a long-lasting habit that enhances your balance, stability, and overall quality of life. Keep in mind that perseverance is crucial and that even the smallest effort contributes to long-term health advantages.

Motivation To Persist For Long-Term Gains

Establishing a balanced weekly routine for physical fitness, especially to enhance stability, balance, and general health, may be challenging. However, the key to success is understanding the long-term advantages and finding the drive to stick to your routine. Here are some constructive ideas and methods to keep you motivated and benefit from your job in the long run.

1. Acknowledge How Crucial Consistency Is

Achieving any fitness objective requires consistency. You will improve the more you practice. Over time, regular exercise enables your body to change and grow. Keep in mind that small, consistent efforts lead to big gains. No matter how small, each workout contributes to your total progress.

2. Instead of Focusing only on the End Goal, Embrace the Journey

Enjoy the trip rather than concentrating just on achieving particular outcomes. Enjoy the journey to improved mobility, balance, and fitness. You may stay motivated and enjoy your program by acknowledging small victories, like finishing a workout or mastering a new exercise.

3. Recognize Your Accomplishments

Note any improvements in your strength, confidence, and balance as you continue to monitor your development. Acknowledging your successes, no matter how small, can boost your drive. Think about keeping a journal or using an app to track your workouts, goals, and post-exercise feelings. Thinking back on your accomplishments may help you remember why you began and inspire you to continue.

4. Locate a Support Network

Seek out a workout partner or surround yourself with encouraging people. Accountability and inspiration can be obtained by discussing your goals and experiences with loved ones, friends, or exercise groups. Support from others could enhance your vacation and motivate you to maintain your objectives.

5. Make Changes to Your Routine

Your needs and interests may change as you get older. To keep things interesting and fun, be open to altering your routine. Find new exercises, courses, or outdoor pursuits that will keep you interested and challenged. Diversity may keep you motivated whether you're taking a community class or trying a new balance exercise.

6. Consider the Advantages That Go Beyond Fitness

Beyond only improving physical health, regular exercise has many other advantages. Increased independence, a decreased chance of falling, and increased confidence in daily duties can all be brought about by improved strength and balance. Additionally, physical activity has been linked to improved mental health, including reduced anxiety, elevated mood, and improved cognitive performance. Your drive to continue your program may increase if you remind yourself of these all-encompassing advantages.

7. Make New Objectives

As you accomplish your initial objectives, think about setting new ones to challenge yourself even more. Your motivation can be boosted by setting new objectives, such as trying a new fitness class, mastering more difficult exercises, or lengthening or intensifying your workouts. You might be inspired to stick with your goals by the sense of accomplishment you get from reaching them.

8. Think about how it will affect your quality of life in the long run

Putting money into your physical well-being today will pay off later. A higher quality of life can result from having better strength and balance, which makes it easier to travel, engage in hobbies, and enjoy activities with loved ones. Seeing the advantages of leading a healthy lifestyle can serve as a powerful incentive to stick to your routine.

9. Be kind to yourself

On this path, treat yourself with kindness. It is quite normal to have days when you are less inspired or encounter difficulties. Practice self-compassion instead of self-criticism. Understand that every effort matters and that taking days off is okay. Concentrate on regaining your focus and reminding yourself of your achievements.

10. Consult a Professional

Consult a fitness expert if you're ever unsure of how to start or wish to enhance your routine. A physical therapist or personal trainer can help you customize your exercise routine to fit your unique requirements and objectives. Their background could boost your self-esteem and guarantee that you're working out safely and correctly.

For seniors, creating and sustaining a healthy weekly routine can have significant long-term advantages. You may design a long-lasting and satisfying fitness path by appreciating the need for consistency, taking pride in your achievements, seeking guidance, and concentrating on holistic changes. Keep in mind that every action you take to improve your health results in a more vibrant, satisfying life. To achieve greater stability, balance, and well-being, embrace the process, stay involved, and relish the journey.

CONCLUSION

As we come to the end of this book, pause to reflect on how much you've learned, practiced, and improved your posture, stability, and balance. You now have a toolkit that will enable you to face every day with a newfound sense of self-assurance, strength, and independence—it's not just workouts.

It takes more than just physical effort to improve your balance. You may accomplish more on this journey with less stress and worry about possible hazards, which enhances your quality of life. You've progressively acquired the abilities needed to address typical challenges faced by seniors, like reduced mobility, the risk of falling, and poor posture, with each chapter. You should have been motivated to prioritize balance in your daily life by the concepts and activities presented in this book, which also offered strategies to help you stay on course as you grow.

Balance training is a lifelong endeavor. Finding balance in real life requires patience and perseverance, just as each chapter of this book gave you useful tactics. Your body's stability is improved by the exercises you've learned, which range from simple sitting activities to more complex standing exercises.

Recall that balancing is a crucial skill that has a direct impact on your self-assurance, independence, and security. The foundation of a healthier life is strengthened when you reaffirm your commitment to performing these exercises regularly. Following your established routines can help you become more stable, reduce your risk of falling, improve your posture, and increase your range of motion—all of which are critical for leading a fulfilling and active life.

Your practice of balancing might have gained additional depth from the breathing techniques chapter. These breathing techniques are crucial for promoting attention and calming the mind, both of which may be quite helpful when performing balancing exercises. You may respond effectively and keep control by synchronizing your breathing and movement, which makes you more present and conscious of the positions and sensations of your body.

Embrace these breathing techniques as a lifelong ability. They can be done anywhere and at any time, whether you're waiting in line, sitting at home, or walking in the park. Breathing can help you maintain your composure, improve your reaction time, and keep your body and mind in sync. Regardless of age or ability, these techniques will support you in keeping your stability and balance as you get older.

You may have noticed that your body's ability to steady, balance, and strengthen itself improved as you advanced through the beginner, intermediate, and expert levels of the exercises. Every step was thoughtfully designed to push and inspire you, enabling you to progress at your speed safely and efficiently. Whether standing or sitting, each exercise level builds on the one before it, enabling you to gradually improve your physical prowess and confidence.

Now that you've reached this milestone, don't be afraid to try new exercises and return to the fundamentals. Even simple exercises done regularly can have a big impact on balance, which is a dynamic concept. The muscles, reflexes, and coordination that support stability are strengthened when you return to these exercises regularly. To keep yourself interested and challenging, switch up your workouts or make small tweaks as your confidence increases.

When you create your own customized balance routine, you have the resources to build a weekly practice that fits your needs, goals, and lifestyle. Instead of seeming like a job, a consistent balance program should feel like an improvement in your life. You might include particular exercises into your everyday duties or warm up with a few workouts in the morning.

Monitoring your development is a great way to stay inspired and understand your progress. From reaching for items on a high shelf to walking confidently in unfamiliar or uneven terrain, even minor adjustments to your balance, mobility, and flexibility can have a big impact on your day-to-day activities. Assess your progress regularly and acknowledge each success, whether it's completing a challenging balance task or maintaining a single-leg stance for a few more seconds.

One of the most crucial elements of any successful exercise regimen is motivation. Remember the many advantages of balancing training, such as a decreased chance of falling, better posture, more stability, and confidence, even when your passion may wane. Every workout you perform is a step toward a safer, more active lifestyle, and you're also increasing your health and quality of life.

Return to the basics when you're feeling unmotivated. To get back into your routine, start with simpler exercises and think about the advantages you've already experienced. Imagine the freedom and mobility that come with having a good balance, and keep in mind that every effort—no matter how small—contributes to the creation of a healthy future. Staying on track can be facilitated by having a support system, which could include friends, family, or an online community.

Balance training has several benefits beyond only reducing the risk of falls. By concentrating on improving your balance, you're making an investment in numerous long-term health advantages. A more active and pleasurable life is a result of improved circulation, increased strength, improved coordination, and increased physiological awareness.

Other fitness components like flexibility and endurance are also enhanced by balance training, which makes it easier to move in a range of settings. You develop the skills and fortitude required to truly enjoy life's adventures with every practice session. The way you manage everyday tasks, travel, hobbies, and relationships with loved ones can all be greatly enhanced over time by these exercises.

Know that you have the resources, knowledge, and support you need to keep getting better at balancing for years to come when you finish this book. You've acquired a set of abilities that you can apply in regular circumstances and modify as you get older. The special ability of balance training to adjust to your evolving demands will help you preserve your stability, self-assurance, and independence for many years to come.

Keep in mind that there is no rush or deadline because this is your trip. Proceed at a pace that feels empowering and comfortable to you. You're moving closer to being a stronger, more resilient version of yourself every day you practice. Celebrate your progress along the way and have faith in your body's capacity to change and evolve.